THE COMPLETE CANCER DIET

COOKBOOK FOR BEGINNERS

A Step-by-Step Guide to Nourishing Whole-Food

Anticancer Recipes for Healing and Wellness

Adam C.

DEDICATION

This book is dedicated to all my Readers

CONTENTS

Introduction

About This Cookbook

Thank you for visiting "The Complete Cancer Diet Cookbook for Beginners: A Step-by-Step Guide to Nourishing Whole-Food Anticancer Recipes for Healing and Wellness." This eBook is going to be your go-to resource for improved health and wellbeing both before and after cancer treatment. It is a thorough resource for individuals who may be navigating the world of cancer and nutrition for the first time, having been carefully designed with novices in mind.

The Role of Nutrition in Cancer Care

The fight against cancer is fierce, and recovery can be difficult. The food you eat, however, is one of your most effective instruments. A crucial part of cancer care is nutrition. An intelligently planned diet can strengthen your immune system, help your body mend itself, and manage adverse effects. During a difficult period, the correct nutrients can boost your energy, lower inflammation, and improve your general quality of life.

We will examine the science of nutrition and cancer treatment in this eBook, illuminating the ways in which different nutrients might enhance your overall health and well-being. We'll talk about the value of selecting whole foods, adopting a plant-based diet, and selecting a diet that suits your individual needs.

How to Use This Guide

We've organized this book to be your dependable travel companion because we want it to be a useful and easy-to-use resource. This eBook is for anybody who wants to learn more about the relationship between nutrition and cancer care, regardless of whether they are a patient, a caregiver, or a worried friend or family member.

We advise you to begin at the beginning and progressively work your way through each chapter in order to get the most out of this book. You'll find insightful information, professional guidance, and, of course, a variety of tasty and nutritious recipes designed to enhance your wellbeing in every department.

You will learn how to prepare anticancer meals step-by-step, how to equip your kitchen with necessary products, and how to plan your meals and regulate portion sizes. We'll also cover how to modify recipes to accommodate particular dietary requirements and deal with the particular difficulties that cancer patient could encounter.

We hope you will make extensive use of this eBook as a reference, using it whenever you are in need of direction or motivation. Taste, nutrition, and convenience of preparation are prioritized in the creation of these dishes, which aim to be both practical and approachable.

Keep in mind that this eBook should not be used in place of medical advice or care. For individualized advice suited to your particular circumstances, always seek the advice of your healthcare practitioner.

With the help of healthy, whole-food anticancer dishes, we are here to assist you on your path to recovery and wellness. Together, let's set out on this life-changing journey and make progress toward a happier, healthier lifestyle.

Chapter 1: Understanding the Basics

1.1 What is Cancer?

A complex and multidimensional set of disorders known as cancer are defined by the body's aberrant cells growing and spreading out of control. It can damage almost any organ or tissue and take on many forms. Cancer is a powerful enemy, but it's important to keep in mind that it's actually a variety of disorders, each with its own distinct features, rather than a single, all-encompassing illness.

When natural processes that control cell growth and division are interfered with, either by genetic changes or by external influences, healthy cells can turn into cancerous ones. These aberrant cells have the potential to infect neighboring tissues or develop tumors over time, impairing the organs' ability to function normally. Metastasis is the process by which cancer spreads to other places of the body if it is not properly treated or managed.

1.2 The Importance of Nutrition

An essential component of cancer care is nutrition. The foods you eat have a significant impact on how the condition is treated and managed. A healthy diet can:

1. Encourage Your Immune System: Relentlessly battling cancer and its aftereffects requires a robust immune system. Foods high in nutrients can strengthen your body's defenses.

2. Give Energy: The physical demands of cancer and its therapies can result in weariness and muscle loss. Eating a balanced diet might help you stay energized.

3. Minimize Inflammation: Prolonged inflammation can aggravate symptoms of cancer and is frequently linked to the disease. Some foods have anti-inflammatory qualities that can reduce pain.

4. Support Healing: Eating foods high in nutrients encourages the regeneration and repair of damaged tissues, which helps the healing process.

5. Boost General Well-Being: Eating a healthy diet can help you live a better life by preserving your energy, controlling side effects, and handling the emotional aspects of your cancer experience.

1.3 Key Nutrients for Cancer Patients

Certain nutrients play a major role in your fight against cancer because of their capacity to promote your overall health and wellbeing. Among these vital nutrients are:

1. Protein: Protein is essential for immune system support, wound healing, and muscle mass maintenance. Lean meats, chicken, fish, legumes, and dairy products are all excellent sources.

2. Antioxidants: Antioxidants, which include selenium and the vitamins C and E, aid in shielding cells from harm brought on by free radicals. Nuts, whole grains, and vibrant fruits and vegetables are good sources of them.

3. Omega-3 Fatty Acids: Due to their anti-inflammatory qualities, omega-3s may be helpful in controlling inflammation and symptoms associated with cancer. Walnuts, flaxseeds, and fatty fish (such as mackerel and salmon) are some of the sources.

4. Fiber: Consuming a lot of fiber can help with weight management, digestion, and the prevention of several types of cancer. Fruits, vegetables, legumes, and whole grains are all great sources of dietary fiber.

5. Micronutrients: Vital vitamins and minerals, such calcium, vitamin D, and folate, are important for sustaining general health and assisting with particular treatment plans. To find out what your specific needs are, speak with your healthcare practitioner.

1.4 Dietary Guidelines for Cancer Patients

Maintaining a balanced diet that fits your unique needs and treatment plan is crucial when coping with cancer. The following general dietary recommendations apply to cancer patients:

1. Adopt a Whole-Foods Diet: The best option for promoting your health is to eat whole, unprocessed foods because they are high in nutrients and devoid of additives.

2. Keep Yourself Hydrated: Staying properly hydrated is essential, particularly if you're having adverse effects like nausea or diarrhea. Drink a lot of water and eat foods high in water content, such as cucumber and watermelon.

3. Keep an eye on portion sizes: It's critical to balance your meals. If you have trouble finishing huge servings, choose smaller, more frequent meals.

4. Adapt to food Restrictions: Develop a nutrition plan that suits your needs in close consultation with a certified dietitian if your treatment calls for any particular food changes.

5. Handle Side Effects: Several cancer therapies may result in unpleasant side effects, such as dysphagia, nausea, or taste alterations. Adjust your diet to lessen these difficulties.

6. Take Note of Your Body: Observe how your body reacts to various meals and modify your diet accordingly. As you travel, your tolerances and preferences might shift.

The first stages towards recovery and wellbeing are learning the fundamentals of cancer, appreciating the role nutrition plays, and identifying necessary nutrients and dietary requirements. We will explore these ideas in more detail in the upcoming chapters, offering helpful guidance, recipes, and resources to support you as you work to enhance your health and quality of life.

Chapter 2: Stocking Your Kitchen

Setting up your kitchen is an essential first step in adopting a cancer-conscious diet. Having a well-stocked kitchen with the appropriate appliances, supplies, and a conscientious purchasing strategy can pave the way for your success in creating healthy whole-food anticancer recipes.

2.1 Essential Kitchen Tools

To make meal preparation easier and more fun, it's a good idea to have a few basic kitchen utensils on available before you start experimenting with anticancer cooking. Here are a few essentials:

1. Cutting Board: When dicing, slicing, and chopping fruits and vegetables, a good cutting board is a need.

2. Knives: For accurate cutting, choose a decent pair of kitchen knives, which should include a chef's knife and a paring knife.

3. Pots and Pans: You can cook a wide range of recipes if you have a selection of pots and pans in various sizes and materials.

4. Baking sheets: Baking sheets are great for making fresh, healthful snacks and roasting veggies.

5. Blender or Food Processor: Blenders and food processors are multipurpose kitchen tools that come in very handy for creating sauces, smoothies, soups, and more.

6. Measuring Cups and Spoons: Keep these in your kitchen to ensure accuracy when following recipes.

7. Mixing Bowls: Having an assortment of mixing bowls in different sizes will improve the efficiency of food preparation.

8. Grater and Zester: Graters and zesters are helpful equipment for zesting citrus fruit, cheese, or spices.

9. Colander: A colander is necessary for washing grains, draining pasta, and rinsing produce.

10. Can Opener: Don't overlook this indispensable gadget for cracking open ingredients from cans.

2.2 Pantry Staples

You can create healthy meals without making frequent excursions to the grocery store if your pantry is well-stocked. Keep the following basic items in your pantry on hand:

1. Whole Grains: Make sure you have enough of oats, brown rice, quinoa, and whole wheat pasta.

2. Canned Beans: High in fiber and protein are beans such kidney beans, chickpeas, and black beans.

3. Tomatoes in a can: Tomatoes work well as a base for stews, sauces, and soups.

4. Broth: Soups and stews can be made with broth vegetable, chicken, or beef.

5. Olive Oil: Extra virgin olive oil is the best option for cooking and spreading over salads.

6. Vinegars: White wine, red wine, and balsamic vinegars give marinades and dressings taste.

7. Herbs and Spices: Adding a range of herbs and spices to your food can enhance its flavor. Think of herbs like turmeric, cumin, thyme, basil, and oregano.

8. Nuts and Seeds: Rich nutrient sources include almonds, walnuts, flaxseeds, and chia seeds.

9. Nut Butter: For a nutritious spread, go for natural, unsweetened nut butter.

10. Honey and Maple Syrup: Use honey and maple syrup sparingly as they are natural sweets.

2.3 Fresh Ingredients

When it comes to cooking against cancer, fresh ingredients are just as important as cabinet staples. Since colorful fruits and vegetables are high in vitamins, minerals, and antioxidants, try to include a range of them in your diet. Consider using the following fresh ingredients:

1. Leafy Greens: Rich in nutrients, spinach, kale, and arugula are great in sautés, smoothies, and salads.

2. Brightly colored vegetables: Bell peppers, carrots, broccoli, and beets give your dishes flavor and nutrition.

3. Berries: Antioxidants abound in raspberries, strawberries, and blueberries.

4. Citrus Fruits: Vitamin C is found in oranges, grapefruits, and lemons.

5. Herbs: You may improve the flavor of your food by adding fresh herbs like cilantro, parsley, and basil.

6. Lean Proteins: For a well-balanced diet, include tofu, fish, poultry, and turkey.

7. Dairy or Dairy Alternatives: You can include dairy-free versions of milk, yogurt, and cheese in your recipes.

2.3 Smart Shopping Tips

When you start your anticancer culinary adventure, remember these wise purchasing suggestions:

1. Plan Your Meals: To cut down on waste and make sure you have everything you need, create a shopping list based on your weekly meal plan.

2. Read Labels: Look for artificial additives, preservatives, and extra sugars on food labels. Select minimally processed products.

3. Purchase in Season: In season produce is sometimes fresher and more reasonably priced.

4. Shop the Periphery: Processed items are usually found in the interior aisles of the grocery store, whereas fresh produce, meats, and dairy are usually found in the outer aisles.

5. Invest in Bulk: To cut costs and minimize packaging waste, think about investing in large quantities of non-perishable goods.

6. Keep Yourself Hydrated: Remember to add water and other healthful drinks to your shopping list.

Equipping your kitchen with necessary appliances, pantry essentials, and fresh foods, along with forming wise buying practices, will put you in a position to quickly and easily cook healthful anticancer meals. We'll look at a number of recipes that can help you on your path to healing and wellbeing in the chapters that follow.

Chapter 3: Breakfast Delights

Having a hearty and filling breakfast gives you the energy and nourishment you need to start the day off well. This chapter will cover a wide range of breakfast options that will please your palate and promote your overall health and wellbeing during your cancer journey.

3.1 Energizing Smoothies

Smoothies are an excellent method to get extra nutrients into your daily routine. They can be easily customized to meet your dietary requirements and taste preferences, and they are quick to prepare. To get you started, try these energy-boosting smoothie recipes:

Berry Blast Smoothie

Ingredients:

- One cup of mixed berries, including blueberries, raspberries, and strawberries
- One mature banana
- 1 cup of leafy spinach
- One-third cup chia seeds

- 1 cup almond milk without sugar

- One tablespoon of optionally sweetened maple syrup or honey

Instructions:

1 In blender, combine all ingredients.

2 Blend till creamy and smooth.

3 After pouring into a glass, savor your smoothie, Berry Blast!

Green Goddess Smoothie

Ingredients:

- One cup of de-stemmed kale leaves

- Half a cucumber, cut into slices and peel

- One green apple, peeled and diced

- 1 tsp freshly squeezed lemon juice

- One-third cup flaxseeds

- One cup of coconut juice

- Cubes of ice (optional)

Instructions:

1 Blend together kale, cucumber, green apple, flaxseeds, lemon juice, and coconut water in a blender.

2 Blend until smooth.

3   If using ice cubes add them and blend once more until thoroughly combined.

4   Pour into a glass, and then savor your smoothie, green goddess!

3.2 Nutrient-Packed Oatmeal

A satisfying and adaptable breakfast choice, oatmeal is a fantastic source of energy and fiber. Try this easy and nutrient-dense oatmeal recipe:

Superfood Oatmeal Bowl

Ingredients:

- Half a cup of traditional oats
- One cup almond milk without sugar and one spoonful chia seeds
- One tsp of hemp seeds
- One tablespoon of almonds, sliced
- One spoonful of maple syrup or honey
- Slices of banana and fresh berries as garnish

Instructions:

1   Combine almond milk and oats in a saucepan. Stirring regularly, simmer over medium heat until the oats are cooked and the mixture thickens.

2   Take off the heat and mix in the sliced almonds, hemp and chia seeds, and maple or honey syrup.

3   Spoon the porridge into a bowl and garnish with banana slices and fresh berries.

4   Savor your superfood oatmeal bowl, loaded with vital minerals and antioxidants!

3.3 Scrumptious Fruit Parfaits

Fruit parfaits are a delicious way to enjoy a range of fruits and textures while also being aesthetically pleasing. This is how to make a delicious fruit parfait:

Layered Fruit Parfait

Ingredients:

- One cup of Greek yogurt, or a dairy-free substitute
- One spoonful of maple syrup or honey
- One-half cup granola

- One cup of chopped fresh mixed fruits (mango, kiwi, and berries)
- Garnish with fresh mint leaves

Instructions:

1. Combine Greek yogurt and honey or maple syrup in a bowl.
2. In serving glasses, layer the bottom with a spoonful of the yogurt mixture.
3. Top with granola and then a layer of mixed fresh fruit.
4. Continue layering until the glass is full, and then add a final layer of fruits.
5. Add some mint leaves as a garnish.
6. To allow the flavors to mingle, refrigerate for a few minutes prior to serving.
7. Savor this delicious layered fruit parfait for a wholesome and revitalizing breakfast!

3.4 Breakfast Wraps and Toasts

Toasts and wraps for breakfast provide countless creative options. They are easy to make and may be tailored with the ingredients of your choice. Here are a few suggestions to get you started when making breakfast:

Avocado Breakfast Wrap

Ingredients:

- One wrap, wholegrain or gluten-free
- 1/2 mashed, ripe avocado
- 1 sliced cooked egg
- Several little spinach leaves
- Add pepper and salt to taste.

Instructions:

1   Over the wrap, equally distribute the mashed avocado.
2   Top the avocado with sliced boiled egg and baby spinach leaves.
3   To taste, add salt and pepper for seasoning.
4   Tightly roll the wrap, and then cut it in half along the diagonal.
5   Savor your filling and healthy avocado breakfast wrap!

Fruit and Nut Toast

Ingredients:

- Two toasted pieces of whole-grain or gluten-free bread
- Two teaspoons of peanut or almond butter
- Strawberries with banana slices

- One tablespoon of finely chopped nuts (pistachios, walnuts, or almonds)
- A drizzle of maple syrup or honey

Instructions:

1 Evenly spread peanut butter or almond butter over the slices of toast.
2 Place strawberries and banana slices on top of the nut butter.
3 After the fruits, scatter chopped nuts on top.
4 For extra sweetness, drizzle with maple syrup or honey.
5 Savor your delicious, crunchy toast with fruit and nuts!

Breakfast is the ideal time to give your body the nourishment and vital nutrients it needs to function. Try out these recipes and feel free to alter them to suit your own tastes. We will look at more meal ideas in the upcoming chapters, so your anticancer diet is not just healthful but also tasty and pleasurable.

Chapter 4: Appetizers and Snacks

A well-rounded anticancer diet goes beyond meals to include filling, wholesome snacks and appetizers that maintain a consistent energy level throughout the day. This chapter will cover a wide range of appetizers and snack options, including homemade popcorn, delectable nut mixes, guilt-free eating, and veggie dips and hummus.

4.1 Veggie Dips and Hummus

Hummus and veggies are a great combination for snacking. They offer an excellent ratio of protein, vitamins, and fiber. In addition to being nutrient-rich, hummus has a smooth, pleasant feel. To get you started, try this easy hummus recipe:

Classic Hummus

Ingredients:

- One can (15 ounces) of rinsed and drained chickpeas
- Triple-spooned tahini
- 2 minced garlic cloves
- Two tsp of lemon juice

- Two tsp of olive oil

- Half a teaspoon of cumin powder

- Add pepper and salt to taste.

- Water as required to get the necessary consistency

- Garnish with olive oil and paprika, if desired.

Instructions:

1 Chickpeas, tahini, garlic, lemon juice, olive oil, and ground cumin should all be combined in a food processor.

2 Add water as necessary to achieve the desired consistency after blending until smooth.

3 To taste, add salt and pepper for seasoning.

4 Garnish with a drizzle of olive oil and a sprinkle of paprika, if you'd like.

5 Serve your traditional hummus with a selection of fresh veggies, such as cherry tomatoes, cucumber slices, and carrot sticks.

4.2 Guilt-Free Snacking

Making decisions about your snacking that are consistent with your anticancer diet is crucial. Choose satiating snacks that are high in nutrients rather than empty calories. Here are some options for guilt-free snacks:

1. Greek Yogurt with Berries: A dish of Greek yogurt with probiotics, antioxidants, and fresh berries drizzled with honey delivers all three.

2. Edamame: A delightful and high-protein snack is made from steamed edamame that has been mildly salted.

3. Apple Slices with Nut Butter: For a filling and well-balanced snack, combine apple slices with peanut or almond butter.

4. Air-Popped Popcorn: Popcorn that has been air-popped and seasoned with a pinch of paprika and nutritional yeast is a tasty and low-calorie snack.

4.3 Tasty Nut Mixes

Nuts are a quick and wholesome snack that is high in protein, heart-healthy fats, and important vitamins and minerals. With a choice of nuts and your favorite seasonings, make your own delicious nut mix. This is a basic recipe to make your own homemade nut mix:

Spiced Nut Mix

Ingredients:

- One cup of mixed nuts, such as cashews, walnuts, and almonds
- One tsp of olive oil
- Half a teaspoon of cumin powder
- One-half tsp paprika
- 1/4 tsp cayenne pepper (modify according to desired level of spiciness)
- Add pepper and salt to taste.

Instructions:

1. Set the oven temperature to 350°F (175°C).
2. Once the mixed nuts are fully coated, put them in a bowl with olive oil, cumin, paprika, cayenne pepper, salt, and pepper.
3. Arrange the seasoned nuts in a single layer on a baking sheet.
4. Roast the nuts for ten to fifteen minutes, or until they are just beginning to roast.
5. Before putting the nuts in an airtight container, let them cool.
6. Savor this tasty, high-protein spiced nut mix as a snack.

4.4 Homemade Popcorn

Whole grain popcorn can be a filling and wholesome snack if it's made with little to no oil or spice. Here's a basic recipe for handmade popcorn:

Herb and Parmesan Popcorn

Ingredients:

- 1/2 cup popcorn kernels
- Two tsp of olive oil
- Parmesan cheese, grated, in 2 tablespoons
- One tsp of dried herbs from Italy
- Add salt to taste.

Instructions:

1 Heat the olive oil in a big pot over medium heat.
2 A few popcorn kernels should be added to the pot before the lid is put on. These kernels indicate that the oil is hot enough when they pop.
3 After the kernels have popped, remove them and add the remaining kernels to the saucepan.
4 To ensure equal heating throughout, place a lid on the pot and give it a gentle shake.

5   Keep shaking the pot from time to time to avoid scorching.

6   Take the saucepan off of the burner when the popping stops.

7   Add salt to taste, dried Italian herbs, and grated Parmesan cheese to the popcorn. For an even coat, toss.

8   Savor your delicious, low-calorie snack of herb and Parmesan popcorn.

A tasty and nutritious addition to your regular routine can be snacks. You can enjoy delectable flavors and maintain your anticancer diet by selecting nutrient-dense foods and homemade snacks. We'll continue to look at ideas and recipes in the next chapters to support your adoption of whole-food anticancer cooking for health and well-being.

Chapter 5: Soups and Salads

This chapter explores a variety of soups and salads that will assist your total well-being on your path to recovery and wellness by nourishing your body, calming your mind, and promoting overall well-being. As adaptable meals that offer vital nutrients, soups and salads are great additions to your anticancer diet.

5.1 Healing Broths

Healing broths are a great option for people receiving cancer treatment since they provide both comfort and nourishment. Because they are easy on the stomach, broths can ease digestive discomfort and nausea. This is an easy recipe for a comforting vegetable stock:

Homemade Vegetable Broth

Ingredients:

- 1 large onion, chopped
- 2 carrots, peeled and chopped
- 2 celery stalks, chopped
- 2 garlic cloves, minced

- cups water
- 1 bay leaf
- Fresh herbs (such as thyme, parsley, or rosemary)
- Salt and pepper to taste

Instructions:

1. In a large pot, heat a bit of olive oil and sauté the onion, carrots, celery, and garlic until they begin to soften.
2. Add the water, bay leaf, and fresh herbs.
3. Bring the mixture to a boil, then reduce the heat and let it simmer for about an hour.
4. Strain the broth to remove the solids and season with salt and pepper to taste.
5. Enjoy your homemade vegetable broth as a soothing and nourishing base for soups or on its own.

5.2 Vibrant Vegetable Soups

A great approach to add a range of nutrients to your diet is with colorful vegetable soups. They provide a filling and cozy supper and are abundant in vitamins, minerals, and antioxidants. This is how to make a traditional minestrone soup:

Minestrone Soup

Ingredients:

- 1 tablespoon olive oil
- 1 onion, chopped
- 2 cloves garlic, minced
- 2 carrots, chopped
- 2 celery stalks, chopped
- 1 zucchini, chopped
- 1 can (14 ounces) diced tomatoes
- 1 can (15 ounces) kidney beans, drained and rinsed
- cups vegetable broth
- 1 cup small pasta (such as ditalini)
- 1 teaspoon dried Italian herbs
- Salt and pepper to taste
- Fresh basil leaves for garnish (optional)

Instructions:

1. In a large pot, heat the olive oil and sauté the onion and garlic until fragrant.
2. Add carrots, celery, zucchini, diced tomatoes, and kidney beans.
3. Pour in the vegetable broth and bring the mixture to a boil.

4   Add pasta and dried Italian herbs, then reduce the heat and let it simmer until the pasta is cooked.

5   Season with salt and pepper to taste.

6   Garnish with fresh basil leaves if desired.

7   Enjoy your homemade Minestrone soup, a hearty and nutrient-rich meal.

5.3 Leafy Green Salads

Salads made with leafy greens are a great way to get vitamins and antioxidants. You may personalize them by adding different fresh veggie toppings. This is a basic recipe for a traditional garden salad:

Classic Garden Salad

Ingredients:

- Mixed leafy greens such as spinach, romaine, and arugula
- Cherry tomatoes, halved
- Cucumber slices
- Red onion, thinly sliced
- Carrot shreds
- Bell pepper, sliced
- Your choice of vinaigrette dressing

Instructions:

1. In a large bowl, combine the mixed leafy greens with cherry tomatoes, cucumber slices, red onion, carrot shreds, and bell pepper.
2. Drizzle your preferred vinaigrette dressing over the salad.
3. Toss to coat the ingredients evenly.
4. Enjoy your classic garden salad as a fresh and nutrient-packed side dish

5.4 Protein-Packed Salads

Salads high in protein provide a filling and healthy dinner. They're perfect for preserving energy and muscle mass while receiving cancer therapy. This is how to make a filling quinoa salad:

Quinoa and Chickpea Salad

Ingredients:

- 1 cup quinoa, rinsed
- 2 cups water
- 1 can (15 ounces) chickpeas, drained and rinsed
- Cherry tomatoes, halved
- Cucumber slices

- Red onion, thinly sliced
- Fresh parsley, chopped
- Lemon vinaigrette dressing
- Salt and pepper to taste

Instructions:

1 In a saucepan, combine quinoa and water. Bring to a boil, then reduce the heat and let it simmer for about 15 minutes or until the quinoa is cooked.
2 Fluff the cooked quinoa with a fork and let it cool.
3 In a large bowl, combine the cooked quinoa with chickpeas, cherry tomatoes, cucumber slices, red onion, and fresh parsley.
4 Drizzle with lemon vinaigrette dressing and season with salt and pepper to taste.
5 Toss to coat all ingredients evenly.

You may get a lot of different nutrients into your diet while keeping your meals light and simple to digest by eating salads and soups. We will continue to look at a range of recipes that complement your anticancer diet and assist you on your path to recovery and wellbeing in the next chapters.

Chapter 6: Main Courses

The focal point of your meals is the main courses, which present a chance to prepare filling, nutrient-dense foods that aid in your recovery and well-being. We will look at many main course possibilities in this chapter, such as dishes with lean protein, vegetarian delicacies, healthful grains and pastas, and delectable seafood concoctions.

6.1 Lean Protein Dishes

During cancer treatment, lean protein sources are crucial for preserving general health and muscle mass. These recipes minimize saturated fats while offering a good amount of protein, vitamins, and minerals. Here's a quick and tasty grilled chicken breast recipe:

Grilled Lemon Herb Chicken Breast

Ingredients:

- 2 boneless, skinless chicken breasts
- 2 tablespoons olive oil
- 2 cloves garlic, minced

- Zest and juice of 1 lemon

- 1 tablespoon fresh rosemary, chopped

- Salt and pepper to taste

Instructions:

1 In a bowl, mix the olive oil, minced garlic, lemon zest, lemon juice, and chopped rosemary.

2 Season the chicken breasts with salt and pepper.

3 Brush the chicken with the lemon herb marinade, making sure it's evenly coated.

4 Preheat the grill to medium-high heat.

5 Grill the chicken for about 6-8 minutes on each side or until the internal temperature reaches 165°F (74°C).

6 Let the chicken rest for a few minutes before slicing.

7 Enjoy your grilled lemon herb chicken breast as a lean and flavorful protein source.

6.2 Vegetarian Delights

A great approach to get a range of plant-based nutrients in your diet is through vegetarian cuisine. They can be delicious and gratifying. This is a wholesome, nutrient-dense stew made

Black Bean and Sweet Potato Stew

Ingredients:

- 2 sweet potatoes, peeled and diced
- 2 cans (15 ounces each) black beans, drained and rinsed
- 1 onion, chopped
- cloves garlic, minced
- 1 can (15 ounces) diced tomatoes
- cups vegetable broth
- 1 teaspoon ground cumin
- 1 teaspoon chili powder
- Salt and pepper to taste
- Fresh cilantro leaves for garnish (optional)

Instructions:

1. In a large pot, sauté the onion and garlic until fragrant.
2. Add the sweet potatoes, black beans, diced tomatoes, vegetable broth, ground cumin, and chili powder.
3. Bring the mixture to a boil, then reduce the heat and let it simmer for about 20-25 minutes, or until the sweet potatoes are tender.
4. Season with salt and pepper to taste.
5. Garnish with fresh cilantro leaves if desired.
6. Enjoy your black bean and sweet potato stew as a hearty and nutritious vegetarian meal.

6.3 Wholesome Grains and Pastas

Pastas and whole grains are great providers of fiber and energy. They might serve as a flexible starting point for your major courses. This is a recipe for whole wheat pasta with roasted veggies that is both healthful and comforting:

Whole Wheat Pasta with Roasted Vegetables

Ingredients:

- ounces whole wheat pasta
- 1 red bell pepper, sliced
- 1 yellow bell pepper, sliced
- 1 zucchini, sliced
- 1 red onion, sliced
- 2 cloves garlic, minced
- 2 tablespoons olive oil
- 1 teaspoon dried Italian herbs
- Salt and pepper to taste
- Grated Parmesan cheese for garnish (optional)

Instructions:

1   Preheat your oven to 400°F (200°C).

2   In a large bowl, toss the sliced bell peppers, zucchini, red onion, and minced garlic with olive oil, dried Italian herbs, salt, and pepper.

3   Spread the seasoned vegetables on a baking sheet and roast for about 20-25 minutes, or until they are tender and slightly caramelized.

4   While the vegetables are roasting, cook the whole wheat pasta according to the package instructions.

5   Drain the pasta and combine it with the roasted vegetables.

6   Season with salt and pepper to taste.

7   Garnish with grated Parmesan cheese if desired.

8   Enjoy your whole wheat pasta with roasted vegetables as a wholesome and satisfying main course.

6.4 Savory Seafood Creations

Omega-3 fatty acids, which are vital for healthy vision and protein, are abundant in seafood. This is a recipe for a tasty and nutritious baked salmon dish:

Baked Lemon Garlic Salmon

Ingredients:

- salmon fillets
- 2 tablespoons olive oil
- 2 cloves garlic, minced
- Zest and juice of 1 lemon
- 1 tablespoon fresh dill, chopped
- Salt and pepper to taste
- Lemon slices for garnish

Instructions:

1. Preheat your oven to 375°F (190°C).
2. In a small bowl, mix the olive oil, minced garlic, lemon zest, lemon juice, and fresh dill.
3. Season the salmon fillets with salt and pepper.
4. Brush the salmon with the lemon garlic marinade.
5. Place the salmon fillets on a baking sheet and add a few lemon slices on top.
6. Bake in the preheated oven for about 15-20 minutes or until the salmon flakes easily with a fork.
7. Enjoy your baked lemon garlic salmon as a savory and heart-healthy seafood dish.

The option to make satiating, nutrient-dense foods that fit your anticancer diet during the main courses is excellent. It is possible to enjoy delectable flavors while promoting your path toward healing and wellbeing, regardless of whether you choose lean protein dishes, vegetarian treats, wholesome grains and pastas, or hearty seafood delicacies. We will go deeper into a range of dishes that are intended to support general health and nourish your body in the next chapters.

Chapter 7: Sides and Accompaniments

Enhancing the taste and nutritional content of your meals is largely dependent on the side dishes and accompaniments you serve. We'll look at many side dishes and accompaniments in this chapter, such as vibrant vegetable sides, grains and legumes, flavorful sauces and dressings, and the advantages of include fermented foods in your anticancer diet.

7.1 Colorful Vegetable Sides

In addition to adding color to your meals, colorful veggies are a great source of vitamins, minerals, and antioxidants. You can cook, steam, or sauté them to make tasty and nourishing sides. A basic recipe for roasted rainbow carrots can be found here:

Roasted Rainbow Carrots

Ingredients:

- 1 bunch of rainbow carrots, peeled and trimmed
- 2 tablespoons olive oil
- 1 teaspoon honey
- 1 teaspoon fresh thyme leaves

- Salt and pepper to taste

Instructions:

1   Preheat your oven to 400°F (200°C).

2   In a large bowl, toss the rainbow carrots with olive oil, honey, fresh thyme leaves, salt, and pepper.

3   Spread the carrots on a baking sheet in a single layer.

4   Roast in the preheated oven for about 25-30 minutes, or until the carrots are tender and slightly caramelized.

5   Enjoy your roasted rainbow carrots as a colorful and nutritious vegetable side.

7.2 Legumes and Grains

Legumes and grains are great providers of complex carbs, protein, and fiber. They can be added to major courses or served as sides. This is a healthy recipe for black bean and quinoa salad:

Quinoa and Black Bean Salad

Ingredients:

- 1 cup quinoa, rinsed
- 2 cups water
- 1 can (15 ounces) black beans, drained and rinsed
- 1 red bell pepper, diced

- 1/2 red onion, finely chopped
- Fresh cilantro leaves, chopped
- Lime vinaigrette dressing
- Salt and pepper to taste

Instructions:

1. In a saucepan, combine quinoa and water. Bring to a boil, then reduce the heat and let it simmer for about 15 minutes or until the quinoa is cooked.
2. Fluff the cooked quinoa with a fork and let it cool.
3. In a large bowl, combine the cooked quinoa with black beans, diced red bell pepper, and finely chopped red onion.
4. Drizzle with lime vinaigrette dressing and season with salt and pepper to taste.
5. Garnish with fresh cilantro leaves.
6. Enjoy your quinoa and black bean salad as a satisfying and nutrient-rich side dish.

7.3 Savory Sauces and Dressings

Dressings and sauces can enhance the flavors of your food and provide a little enjoyment that is guilt-free. You can choose the ingredients and make delectable sides when you make your own. This is how to make a basic balsamic vinaigrette dressing:

Balsamic Vinaigrette Dressing

Ingredients:

- 1/4 cup balsamic vinegar
- 1/2 cup extra virgin olive oil
- 1 clove garlic, minced
- 1 teaspoon Dijon mustard
- 1 teaspoon honey
- Salt and pepper to taste

Instructions:

1. In a bowl, whisk together balsamic vinegar, minced garlic, Dijon mustard, honey, salt, and pepper.
2. While whisking, slowly drizzle in the extra virgin olive oil until the dressing is emulsified.
3. Adjust the seasoning to taste.
4. Use your homemade balsamic vinaigrette dressing to enhance the flavor of your salads, vegetables, or other dishes.

7.4 Fermented Foods

Probiotic-rich fermented foods can help maintain a healthy gut micro biome. They support healthy digestion and general health. Including them in your diet can be delicious and beneficial. Here's a basic recipe for making sauerkraut at home:

Homemade Sauerkraut

Ingredients:

- 1 medium cabbage, finely shredded
- 1 1/2 tablespoons sea salt

Instructions:

1 In a large bowl, combine the shredded cabbage and sea salt.

2 Massage the cabbage and salt together for a few minutes until the cabbage begins to release its juices.

3 Pack the cabbage tightly into a clean glass jar or a fermentation crock.

4 Ensure the cabbage is submerged under its own juices.

5 Cover the jar with a lid or a clean cloth secured with a rubber band.

6 Allow the sauerkraut to ferment at room temperature for 1-2 weeks, depending on your taste preference.

7 Once it reaches the desired level of tanginess, store it in the refrigerator.

8 Enjoy your homemade sauerkraut as a probiotic-rich accompaniment to your meals.

Enhancing the nutritional value and flavor of your meals can be achieved through the addition of sides and accompaniments. These accompaniments, which can include colorful vegetable sides, grains and legumes, savory sauces and dressings, or fermented foods, can support you in keeping a balanced and healthful anticancer diet. We'll keep looking at recipes and concepts to help you on your path to wellness in the upcoming chapters.

Chapter 8: Sweet Treats

It is possible to indulge your sweet tooth and follow an anticancer diet at the same time. This chapter will cover a range of sweet treats that will satiate your sweet tooth without sacrificing your commitment to health and recovery. There are lots of options to enjoy, ranging from guilt-free desserts and fruit-based treats to baking with health in mind and refreshing frozen desserts.

8.1 Guilt-Free Desserts

Desserts that don't make you feel guilty can be decadent without going overboard with sugar and bad fats. These sweets are full of flavor and thoughtful of your well-being. A recipe for energizing chocolate protein balls can be found here:

Chocolate Protein Balls

Ingredients:

- 1 cup rolled oats
- 1/2 cup almond butter
- 1/4 cup honey or maple syrup
- 1/4 cup unsweetened cocoa powder

- 2 tablespoons chocolate protein powder

- 1/2 teaspoon vanilla extract

- A pinch of salt

- Optional add-ins: chopped nuts, seeds, or dried fruit

Instructions:

1. In a bowl, combine rolled oats, almond butter, honey or maple syrup, cocoa powder, chocolate protein powder, vanilla extract, and a pinch of salt.

2. If desired, add in chopped nuts, seeds, or dried fruit for extra texture and flavor.

3. Mix until all the ingredients are well combined.

4. Form the mixture into small balls and place them on a baking sheet.

5. Refrigerate for at least 30 minutes to set.

6. Enjoy your chocolate protein balls as a nutritious and energy-boosting dessert.

8.2 Fruit-Based Treats

Fruit-based treats are a great way to satiate your sweet tooth and reap the health benefits of fruits' vitamins and antioxidants. Here's a recipe for a refreshing and fruity pineapple sorbet:

Pineapple Sorbet

Ingredients:

- cups fresh pineapple chunks
- 1/4 cup honey or maple syrup
- 2 tablespoons freshly squeezed lime juice
- 1/4 cup water
- Fresh mint leaves for garnish (optional)

Instructions:

1 Place the fresh pineapple chunks in a blender or food processor.

2 Add honey or maple syrup and freshly squeezed lime juice.

3 Blend until smooth.

4 Add water gradually to achieve your desired sorbet consistency.

5 Transfer the mixture to a freezer-safe container and freeze for a few hours, stirring occasionally to prevent ice crystals from forming.

6 Once the sorbet has reached the desired texture, scoop and garnish with fresh mint leaves if desired.

7 Enjoy your homemade pineapple sorbet as a refreshing and fruit-based delicacy.

8.3 Baking with Health in Mind

Baking with health in mind involves using nutritious ingredients while reducing sugar and unhealthy fats. Here's a recipe for whole wheat banana bread:

Whole Wheat Banana Bread

Ingredients:

- 2 cups whole wheat flour
- 1 teaspoon baking soda
- 1/4 teaspoon salt
- ripe bananas, mashed
- 1/4 cup honey or maple syrup
- 1/4 cup unsweetened applesauce
- 1/4 cup Greek yogurt
- 2 eggs
- 1 teaspoon vanilla extract
- 1/2 cup chopped nuts or chocolate chips (optional)

Instructions:

1 Preheat your oven to 350°F (175°C) and grease a loaf pan.
2 In a bowl, whisk together whole wheat flour, baking soda, and salt.

3   In another bowl, combine mashed bananas, honey or maple syrup, applesauce, Greek yogurt, eggs, and vanilla extract.

4   Gradually add the dry ingredients to the wet ingredients and mix until well combined.

5   If desired, fold in chopped nuts or chocolate chips.

6   Pour the batter into the prepared loaf pan.

7   Bake in the preheated oven for about 50-60 minutes or until a toothpick inserted into the center comes out clean.

8   Allow the banana bread to cool before slicing.

9   Enjoy your whole wheat banana bread as a health-conscious and satisfying dessert.

8.4 Refreshing Frozen Desserts

A delicious way to satisfy your sweet craving and stay cool is by indulging in frozen desserts. This is how to make a cool, creamy mango frozen yogurt:

Frozen Mango Yogurt

Ingredients:

- Three cups frozen mango chunks
- Half cups Greek yogurt
- 1/4 cup honey or maple syrup

- One teaspoon vanilla extract

- Fresh mint leaves for garnish (optional)

Instructions:

1   In a blender or food processor, combine frozen mango chunks, Greek yogurt, honey or maple syrup, and vanilla extract.

2   Blend until smooth and creamy.

3   Transfer the mixture to a freezer-safe container and freeze for a few hours, stirring occasionally to maintain a creamy texture.

4   Once the frozen yogurt reaches the desired consistency, scoop and garnish with fresh mint leaves if desired.

5   Enjoy your homemade mango frozen yogurt as a creamy and refreshing dessert.

You can include sweets in your anticancer diet as long as you make thoughtful decisions that put your health and wellbeing first. There are many methods to sate your sweet tooth while advancing your path to healing and wellbeing, whether you choose guilt-free sweets, fruit-based treats, baking with health in mind, or cool frozen desserts. We will continue to look at ideas and recipes in the next chapters to support you in adopting a healthy whole-food anticancer diet.

Chapter 9: Beverages

Staying properly hydrated is critical to your overall health and well-being and will help you on your path to recovery and wellness. We'll look at a variety of drinks in this chapter that can help you stay nourished and hydrated while following your anticancer diet. There are lots of delicious options to pick from, such as nutrient-rich smoothies, energizing mock tails, and herbal teas and infusions.

9.1 Hydration for Healing

Throughout your cancer journey, it's imperative that you stay well hydrated. It facilitates healthy physical processes, aids with digestion, and removes toxins from the body. To be well hydrated, it's crucial to drink a range of liquids, and the decisions you make can have a big influence on your health.

Do not forget to stay hydrated during the day. Smoothies, mocktails, and herbal teas can all help you meet your daily hydration requirements while providing extra nourishment. Pay attention to your body and choose hydrated foods that complement your anticancer diet when you feel thirsty.

9.2 Herbal Teas and Infusions

Herbal infusions and teas have numerous health advantages in addition to being reassuring. They can give antioxidants, ease gastrointestinal distress, and encourage relaxation. Here are some alternatives for herbal teas and infusions to think about:

1. Tea made with ginger and turmeric: Both spices have anti-inflammatory qualities that can aid in digestion and reduce nausea. Slices of fresh ginger and turmeric should be steeped in boiling water, and a little honey should be added for sweetness.

2. Infusion of chamomile: The relaxing and anti-inflammatory properties of chamomile tea are well-known. A calming and caffeine-free beverage can be made by steeping dried chamomile flowers in hot water.

3. Peppermint Tea: This invigorating beverage has a cooling taste and aids in the relief of digestive problems. A delicious and calming cup of tea can be made by steeping peppermint leaves in hot water.

9.3 Nutrients-Rich Smoothies

An easy and adaptable approach to include a range of nutrients in your diet is through smoothies. They can be customized to meet your dietary requirements and taste preferences. This is how to make a smoothie for a green detox:

Green Detox Smoothie

Ingredients:

- One cup of kale or spinach
- Half a cucumber
- One-half green apple
- 1/2 juiced lemon
- A half-inch-long slice of raw ginger
- One cup coconut water or water
- Cubes of ice (optional)
- Taste-tested honey or maple syrup (optional)

Instructions:

1. Place spinach or kale, cucumber, green apple, lemon juice, fresh ginger, and water in a blender.
2. Blend until smooth. If you prefer a thicker consistency, add ice cubes.

3. If you'd like a touch of sweetness, you can add honey or maple syrup to taste.

4. Enjoy your green detox smoothie as a nutrient-packed and refreshing beverage.

9.4 Refreshing Mocktails

Mocktails are delightfully flavorful non-alcoholic beverages without any alcohol. They can be an enjoyable and revitalizing method to relax or have fun. This is how to make a spicy virgin mojito:

Virgin Mojito

Ingredients:

- 1/2 lime, cut into wedges
- 8-10 fresh mint leaves
- 1 tablespoon honey or maple syrup
- Club soda
- Ice cubes

Instructions:

1. In a glass, muddle lime wedges and fresh mint leaves together.
2. Add honey or maple syrup and stir to combine.

3. Fill the glass with ice cubes.

4. Top off with club soda.

5. Garnish with a sprig of fresh mint and a lime wedge.

6. Enjoy your virgin mojito as a refreshing and zesty mocktail.

A satisfying and pleasurable addition to your anticancer diet might be beverages. Smoothies that are high in nutrients, herbal teas and infusions, or cool mocktails can all assist you in staying properly hydrated and advancing your path to health and well-being. We will continue to look at recipes and ideas to support you in adopting a whole-food anticancer diet for your health in the upcoming chapters.

Chapter 10: Meal Planning and Portion Control

Maintaining a nutritious whole-food anticancer diet requires careful meal planning and plate balancing. This chapter will include portion control techniques, meal prep hacks to make cooking more efficient, methods for preparing balanced and nutritional meals, and advice on customizing the recipes to suit your own requirements.

10.1 Balancing Your Plate

A plate that is balanced gives you a range of nutrients and guarantees that your meal is well-rounded. To do this, take into account the following recommendations:

1. Vegetables Should Make Up Half of Your Plate: Vegetables are a great source of antioxidants, vitamins, and minerals. You can guarantee that you are getting the necessary nutrients by having a colorful assortment of veggies make up half of your plate.

2. Add Lean Proteins: To maintain muscular health and give long-lasting energy, include lean protein sources including fish, chicken, lentils, and tofu.

3. Incorporate Nutritious Grains: Nutritious grains, such as brown rice, quinoa, and whole wheat pasta, provide fiber and complex carbs that promote sustained energy and satiety.

4. Include Healthy Fats: To add healthy fats that enhance nutrient absorption and general wellbeing, incorporate nuts, avocados, and olive oil into your meals.

5. Reduce the Amount of Processed Foods: Refined and processed foods are sometimes heavy in sugar, bad fats, and additives.

6. Remain Hydrated: To stay properly hydrated, don't forget to consume water and other wholesome drinks.

10.2 Meal Prep Tips

Organizing your meals can improve the efficiency, enjoyment, and manageability of your anticancer diet. Consider the following meal preparation advice:

1. Plan Your Meals: Make a weekly food plan taking into

account your dietary preferences and constraints.

2. Make a Shopping List: To make sure you have all the ingredients you need, make a shopping list based on your meal plan.

3. Cooking in bulk: Prepare bigger amounts of cereals, meats, and veggies, then split them out and keep them in containers that fit your needs for the week.

4. Prep Fresh Ingredients: Prepare fresh ingredients by washing, chopping, and preparing them so that they are ready to use for quick meal preparation or as snacks.

5. Employ Reusable Containers: To store prepared foods and ingredients, make an investment in reusable containers. This keeps your food fresh and minimizes waste.

6. Portion Control: Pay attention to how much food you put in your mouth, especially when it comes to high-calorie foods.

10.3 Portion Control Strategies

To make sure you're getting the correct quantity of nutrients without going overboard, portion control is crucial. The following are some methods for portion control:

1. Use Smaller Dishes: Using smaller dishes might aid in the organic reduction of portion sizes.

2. Mindful Eating: Be aware of your body's signals of hunger and fullness. Savor each piece of food, eat slowly, and stop eating when you're full.

3. Protein Portion: Lean protein portions typically measure roughly the same size as a deck of cards. Try to have protein on one-quarter of your plate.

4. Grains and Carbs: You can put grains or carbohydrates on the last part of your plate. Typically, a single serving is the size of your fist.

5. Fill Up on Vegetables: To give your meal more substance without adding too many calories, load up on vegetables.

6. Snack Wisely: When having a snack, divide up a dish instead of eating it straight out of the container.

7. Steer clear of distractions: Eating in front of a computer or TV might result in mindless overindulgence in food. Aim to eat at a table free from interruptions.

10.4 Adapting the Recipes to Your Needs

Dietary requirements and tastes vary from person to person. You can modify the recipes in this cookbook to meet your unique needs. Here are some criteria for adaptation:

1. Allergies and Dietary limitations: Use items that are suitable for you if you have any allergies or dietary limitations. For example, if you have gluten intolerance, use gluten-free pasta.

2. Caloric Requirements: Modify serving sizes and component amounts to satisfy your calorie requirements. It might be necessary to adjust the scales for some recipes.

3. Taste Preferences: You are welcome to change the recipes to fit your own tastes. Add extra spices or chili peppers to your food if you like it hotter.

4. Texture Preferences: Blend or puree your food to make it simpler to swallow if you have trouble with a particular texture because of medical treatments.

5. Meal Timing: You can modify recipes to suit your chosen meal timings based on your appetite and treatment plan.

Keep in mind that your path to health and wellbeing is unique to you, and it's crucial that the decisions you make reflect your requirements and objectives. You can design an anticancer diet that is both healthy and sustainable for you by modifying the recipes to fit your specific needs.

Chapter 11: Special Considerations

There are a number of unique factors to consider while catering to the dietary requirements of cancer patients. These issues will be covered in detail in this chapter, along with dietary restrictions and allergies, preparing meals for a loved one undergoing cancer, creating recipes that are specific to their symptoms, and the significance of speaking with a healthcare professional.

11.1 Dietary Restrictions and Allergies

Patients with cancer may need to pay close attention to any dietary restrictions or allergies they may have. Here are some crucial things to think about:

1. Allergies: Take note of any dietary sensitivities or allergies the person may have. Common allergies including nuts, shellfish, and gluten may be among them. To avoid using problematic items, always read labels before modifying recipes.

2. Medication Interactions: Certain foods and medications used to treat cancer may interact with one another. To make sure there are no negative interactions between the patient's food and treatment, speak with a healthcare professional or dietitian.

3. Texture Modifications: Individuals may require their food to be blended, pureed, or presented in a certain texture depending on the side effects of their medication. Make sure the cuisine is appetizing as well as safe.

4. Hydration: Individuals receiving cancer therapy may notice taste alterations or swallowing difficulties. In these situations, coming up with tasty and hydrating dishes becomes essential.

5. Caloric and Nutrient Requirements: Depending on their treatment stage, patients may need to consume varied amounts of calories and nutrients. Work together with nutritionists or healthcare professionals to match recipes to certain nutritional requirements.

11.2 Cooking for a Loved One with Cancer

Making meals for a loved one battling cancer can be a powerful way to show support and compassion. Here are some pointers to think about:

1. Communication is essential: It must be honest and open. Inquire about the person's dietary choices, what they can and cannot eat, and any particular wants or aversions they may have.

2. Flexibility: Be ready to modify your meal to suit each person's requirements. To accommodate their preferences, this can entail preparing different meals, adjusting textures, or switching up ingredients.

3. Emotional Support: Meal preparation can be emotionally exhausting for the patient as well as the caregiver. Provide tolerance, understanding, and emotional support during this trying time.

4. Meal Variety: To avoid food fatigue and provide the patient a range of flavors and textures to savor, prepare a variety of dishes.

5. Small Frequent Meals: An appetite may be affected by cancer treatment. To guarantee proper nourishment, think about offering meals and snacks more frequently and in smaller portions.

6. Hydration: Encourage people to stay hydrated and offer options for doing so, as this is important during cancer treatment.

11.3 Recipes for Specific Symptoms

Mouth sores to nausea are just a few of the symptoms that cancer and its treatments can produce. Making mealtimes more comfortable can be achieved by modifying dishes to accommodate certain problems. Here are some ideas for recipes:

1. Nausea: You can get rid of nausea by drinking ginger tea, having broths, and eating simple, easily digested foods like applesauce and rice.

2. Dry Mouth: Foods that are moist and tasty, like stews and soups, can make a person feel less parched.

3. Mouth Sores: People who suffer from mouth sores often find relief from soft, comforting meals like smoothies, yoghurt, and mashed potatoes.

4. Weight Loss: People who are having trouble losing weight can benefit from high-calorie, high-protein dishes like protein drinks and calorie-dense soups.

5. Digestive Problems: Rice, steamed veggies, and poached chicken are examples of light, easily digested foods that are easier on the digestive tract.

11.4 Consultation with a Healthcare Provider

Finally, it is imperative to stress that seeking the counsel and direction of a medical professional or certified dietician is always advisable. They are able to handle any dietary or medical problems and offer customized recommendations.

1. Speak with a Dietitian: Based on the patient's unique requirements, preferences, and stage of treatment, a registered dietitian can develop a personalized nutritional plan.

2. Medication and Treatment Considerations: Make sure the patient's diet and treatment regimens work together. Medication and some foods and supplements may interfere.

3. Frequent Check-Ins: Keep an eye on the patient's nutritional state and modify the diet plan as necessary by consulting dietitians and healthcare professionals on a regular basis.

4. Handling Weight Changes: Seek advice on how to manage the patient's weight changes through nutrition and food if they undergo a substantial amount of weight gain or loss.

5. Supportive treatment: There may be more possibilities for both integrative and supportive treatment. These cover a range of well-being-related services, such as massage, acupuncture, and counseling.

In conclusion, it is critical to address unique factors related to the nutritional requirements of cancer patients. A complete approach can have a big impact on the patient's well-being and healing process, whether it involves catering to dietary restrictions and allergies, cooking for a loved one who has cancer, customizing recipes for specific symptoms, or consulting with healthcare specialists and nutritionists. When it comes to providing dietary support for cancer patients, tailored care, empathy, and open communication should always come first.

Chapter 12: Lifestyle and Wellness

Well-being and healing transcend your plate. We'll look at the key elements of a holistic approach to well-being in the context of cancer treatment in this last chapter. This entails embracing mindful eating techniques, moving "Beyond the Plate," realizing the importance of exercise in cancer treatment, and fostering emotional wellbeing.

12.1 Beyond the Plate

A healthy, whole-food anticancer diet is essential, but it's just one component of the picture. A holistic approach to wellness and healing takes into account a number of factors, including:

1. Stress management: Excessive stress can have a detrimental effect on your general health. Using stress-reduction methods like deep breathing, mindfulness, or meditation can help you deal with cancer's problems more effectively.

2. Sleep: For healing and recuperation, getting enough good sleep is crucial. Establish a regular sleep schedule and create a cozy sleeping environment to aid in your body's natural healing processes.

3. Toxin Reduction: You can improve your health by limiting your exposure to environmental toxins like chemicals and pollutants. Make thoughtful decisions and use eco-friendly cleaning supplies in your daily life.

4. Community and Support: Getting emotional help from loved ones, friends, or support groups can be extremely important to your recovery process. Never be afraid to ask for help when you need it.

12.2 Mindful Eating

The act of focusing entirely on the dining experience from the tastes and textures of your food to your body's feelings is known as mindful eating. This strategy can improve your general wellbeing and help you have a healthy relationship with food.

1. Present-Moment Awareness: Pay attention to the here and now as you eat. Keep your eyes off of distractions like television and smartphones and focus on the flavors, colors, and aromas of your cuisine.

2. Savor Every Bite: Chew each bite slowly. Chew mindfully, appreciating the flavor and consistency of your food. This may facilitate fullness and digestion.

3. Cues for Hunger and Fullness: Pay attention to the cues your body sends forth. Even if there is food left on your plate, you should only eat when you are hungry and quit when you are full.

4. Non-Judgmental Awareness: Have a non-judgmental attitude when eating. Treat yourself with kindness and stop berating yourself for your dietary decisions.

12.3 Exercise and Cancer Care

Exercise is important for cancer patients since it has several physical and mental health advantages. Prior to starting or altering an exercise regimen, always check with your healthcare practitioner, but take into account the following:

1. Strengthening the Body: Throughout cancer treatment, regular exercise can help preserve physical health in general and muscle strength and mobility in particular.

2. Mood Boosting: Research has indicated that physical activity can lower anxiety and sadness, elevate mood, and improve overall well-being.

3. Boosting Immunity: Engaging in physical activity can enhance your body's defenses against disease and strengthen your immune system.

4. Weariness Management: Exercise can help reduce cancer-related weariness and boost general energy levels, despite the fact that this may seem paradoxical.

5. Tailored Exercise Programs: Consult a physician, physical therapist, or fitness expert to develop a customized exercise program that meets your objectives and present state of health.

12.4 Emotional Well-being

During your cancer journey, maintaining your mental well-being is crucial to your overall health. The following tactics can help you maintain your emotional well-being:

1. Therapy and Counseling: If you're having emotional

difficulties, you might want to think about getting help from a therapist or counselor who focuses on cancer-related concerns.

2. Mind-Body Techniques: Techniques like tai chi, yoga, and meditation help promote emotional balance and a sensation of peace.

3. Support Networks: Make contact with networks of others going through comparable struggles or support groups. It might be healing to talk about your emotions and experiences.

4. Creativity and Self-Expression: Creating art, music, or writing are examples of creative endeavors that can serve as a healthy emotional release.

5. Positive Affirmations: To improve your emotional wellbeing, make self-compassion and positive affirmations a daily part of your routine.

Keep in mind that dealing with cancer is an extremely personal experience. You may take care of your mental and emotional health in addition to your physical health by adopting a holistic approach to wellness that goes beyond the plate. Throughout this difficult path, remember to be kind to yourself, ask for help when you need it, and take the time to treasure the moments of happiness and connection that can occur. You have a unique road to wellness and healing, and by taking a holistic approach, you'll be better able to handle the challenges along the way with resilience and grace.

Chapter 13: Resources and References

This final chapter of "The Complete Cancer Diet Cookbook for Beginners" provides a valuable list of resources and references to further support your journey toward healing and wellness. These resources include additional reading materials, helpful organizations and websites, and an index of all the recipes featured in the cookbook.

13.1 Additional Reading

Cancer: The Emperor of All Maladies by Siddhartha Mukherjee: This comprehensive book provides an in-depth exploration of the history and science of cancer, offering a profound understanding of the disease.

1. Radical Remission: Surviving Cancer against All Odds by Kelly A. Turner: This book discusses the stories of individuals who achieved radical remission, highlighting nine key factors that played a role in their healing.

2. Anticancer: A New Way of Life by David Servan-Schreiber, MD, PhD: A groundbreaking book that explores the role of diet and lifestyle in cancer prevention and healing.

3. The Cancer-Fighting Kitchen by Rebecca Katz and Mat Edelson: Filled with nourishing recipes, this cookbook is a wonderful resource for those seeking to support their health through diet.

13.2 Helpful Organizations and Websites

1. American Cancer Society (ACS) - www.cancer.org: The ACS is a reliable source for cancer information, research, and support services.

2. National Cancer Institute (NCI) - www.cancer.gov: A comprehensive resource for cancer research, clinical trials, and treatment information.

3. Cancer Care - www.cancercare.org: Cancer Care provides free support services to help those affected by cancer manage the practical and emotional challenges of the disease.

4. World Cancer Research Fund (WCRF) - www.wcrf.org: WCRF is a leading authority on cancer prevention research and

offers valuable information on diet and lifestyle.

5. American Institute for Cancer Research (AICR) - www.aicr.org: AICR is dedicated to advancing cancer research and educating the public about the importance of diet, nutrition, and cancer prevention.

6. Cancer.Net - www.cancer.net: Cancer.Net offers physician-approved information on cancer types, treatment options, and practical advice for living with cancer.

About the Author

Dr. Adam C. stands as a beacon of inspiration in the fields of medicine, nutrition, and self-help, with a remarkable journey that exemplifies the transformative power of healthy living. Armed with a professional master's degree in health nutrition and years of experience, Dr. C. has become a guiding light for individuals seeking to embrace vibrant well-being and lead happier lives.

From an early age, Dr. C. navigated through a myriad of health challenges that ranged from genetic predispositions to the pitfalls of unhealthy eating. His personal struggle ignited a flame of determination within him, one that was fueled by the belief that the human body possesses an incredible ability to heal and rejuvenate through the right nourishment. Through steadfast dedication, Dr. C. managed to conquer his own ailments and emerged as a living testament to the transformative potential of a well-balanced lifestyle.

What sets Dr. Adam C. apart is his rich tapestry of experiences, having been deeply immersed in groundbreaking research in health food and diet-related domains. His quest to uncover the hidden treasures of nutrients within our meals has led to groundbreaking revel actions that empower individuals to extract the maximum benefit from their dietary choices. Dr. C.'s research has not only contributed to the scientific community but has also served as a roadmap for countless individuals striving to optimize their health.

However, it is not just Dr. C.'s academic prowess that has touched lives it is his unparalleled compassion and empathy that truly make him a beacon of hope. His personal journey of triumph over adversity infuses his guidance with an authentic understanding of the challenges his readers and patients face. Dr. C. doesn't just prescribe nutritional plans; he fosters a deep connection with his audience, instilling in them the confidence to embark on their own transformative journeys.

Dr. Adam C.'s holistic approach reaches beyond the confines of traditional medicine. His insights have translated into self-help resources that empower individuals to take charge of their wellness narrative. His words resonate on paper as they do in person, making his books not mere guides, but trusted companions on the path to vitality.

In the realm of health and nutrition, Dr. C. shines as a true luminary. His core strengths lie in his ability to synthesize complex scientific findings into practical, actionable advice that individuals from all walks of life can seamlessly integrate into their routines. Dr. C.'s legacy is not just a collection of breakthroughs; it is a testament to the extraordinary potential that lies within each of us to overcome obstacles and embrace a life brimming with health, happiness, and fulfillment.

As an experienced doctor, passionate nutritionist, and empathetic author, Dr. Adam C. continues to transform lives, showing us that the journey to a healthier, happier existence is within our grasp, waiting to be unlocked through the power of informed choices and unwavering determination.

www.ingramcontent.com/pod-product-compliance
Lightning Source LLC
Chambersburg PA
CBHW050838260726

48660CB00006B/2318